My Heart Will Go On Singing

by

Danny Daniels

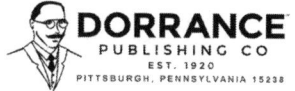

The contents of this work, including, but not limited to, the accuracy of events, people, and places depicted; opinions expressed; permission to use previously published materials included; and any advice given or actions advocated are solely the responsibility of the author, who assumes all liability for said work and indemnifies the publisher against any claims stemming from publication of the work.

·

All Rights Reserved
Copyright © 2023 by Danny Daniels

No part of this book may be reproduced or transmitted, downloaded, distributed, reverse engineered, or stored in or introduced into any information storage and retrieval system, in any form or by any means, including photocopying and recording, whether electronic or mechanical, now known or hereinafter invented without permission in writing from the publisher.

Dorrance Publishing Co
585 Alpha Drive
Pittsburgh, PA 15238
Visit our website at www.dorrancebookstore.com

ISBN: 979-8-88812-119-1
eISBN: 979-8-88812-619-6

FOREWORD

In 1958 an old Texas cowboy wrote a song by the title "Until Then." This song is also referred to as "My heart can sing when I pause to remember." Well, not only is it one of my favorites, but that is exactly what this book is about: remembering what God has done for me over the past thirty years and how he has healed my heart. I am alive today to tell you that until I see my Savior face to face, my heart will go on singing of his goodness, his love, and his faithfulness to one who surely does not deserve it.

Chapter 1

My name is Danny, and I have just celebrated my 72nd birthday in July 2022. I am not a writer; I am a construction worker. I can build you a house, but writing a book is certainly out of my field. Also, anyone that knows me is aware that I have been a "heart patient" since I was thirty-eight years old and have had numerous close calls with death because of my defective heart. Some of you may have even asked "Is he still around?" due to past reports of various heart procedures, surgeries, and episodes. The answer to that question is YES! I am here only because of the goodness of my God and His divine healing power. In February 2019, I had a major heart surgery where I not only experienced my life being changed physically but also spiritually. Because of this divine encounter with the Holy Spirit, I am compelled to write "my story" even if this story is just for me.

While conversing with my psychiatrist earlier this year about how God had intervened in my life so many times, I was reminded of the close calls with death I had experienced but survived due to the intervention of my great God. At that time the psychiatrist casually made the statement that I should write these events down. That way I would never forget them and also be able to share with others about the divine plan that HE has for each of us. I want to share also about the healing power of God for my body, but more than that is how I was changed spiritually. Let me interject here: He desires to change us all. His plan is so perfect for us, and His will is that we would see ourselves as HE sees us. After leaving her office, I began to think of the assignment she had given me. I mentally started rehearsing the past thirty plus years. Before I knew it, I was "pecking" away on my ipad trying to put those events on paper. This writing is the result of what has transpired in my life to the best of my knowledge. I have not written any of this for sympathy or attention to Danny. I have one goal in mind and that is to give TOTAL GLORY and HONOR to GOD for the miracles HE has performed in my life. As you read my poorly written account of the events of my heart journey, please join me in worshiping the KING of KINGS and LORD of LORDS for HIS continuing faithfulness to a hard headed young man who realizes today that his "steps" have been ordered by the Lord. Why me? I will have to get that answer when I get to Heaven. His love for me has surpassed my ability to say, think, or understand. I have failed God so much. My scars are more than I can ever tell. I can only wonder WHY HE LOVES ME SO. The reason for me writing this book is to let you know how much HE has done for me, and how much HE loves you. What HE did for me, He will do for you. You are the apple of his eye. I believe if you seek Jesus, you will find HIM. Oh, the joy, love, and peace you will have when you do. So...until we see Him face to face, let our hearts "go on singing."

Chapter 2

After college in 1972, Peggy, my wife of fifty-one years, and I began working in various churches part time as assistant pastors and worship leaders. We really felt God calling us into ministry; however, nothing ever opened up for us, and we always found ourselves part time. I sought the Lord about this, and I felt that maybe I was to continue in the construction field. Construction came easy for me...it was natural since I had been taught as a young boy to work in this field. I dedicated myself to building, and I certainly saw the blessings of God on my efforts. Yes, there were ups and downs, but God always brought us through any obstacles that we may have faced. Peggy was teaching school; I was building. We were working in the local church. We were never 100% in either field. Yes, we had asked for God to open a full time door. It did not happen so it was just as it was. We would always be part time in whatever job we had. I can honestly say in my heart that I did not have total satisfaction that I was in the perfect will of God. As I look back, I can tell you that God got the short end of my service. Today, I see that clearly, but HE did not cast me away or give up on me. It would be during the next thirty years that I would need HIS intervention in my life because of a "bad heart." He would always be present.

Chapter 3

My health journey has had several definite stops and many times it seemed that life was over for me, but God always brought me through each one. My first scare was in 1989 when we were living and working in Lakeland, Florida. I was working in construction building residential homes. Out of the blue, I experienced severe chest pains and found myself one afternoon in Lakeland General Hospital. I had never had any chest pains prior to this so I was very much concerned knowing that "heart problems" were a DNA "thing" in the

Daniels' family.

After meeting with several doctors and running various tests, a heart catheterization was scheduled the next morning. The doctors discovered two blocked arteries and opened them during this procedure. I stayed in the hospital two nights and before I knew it, I was back to work. I felt great, and life was wonderful. God had allowed my heart problem to be resolved so that I could carry on with my life. As I reflect now on this time, this was the beginning of his intervention in my "heart journey." I was oblivious to his working, and today I feel so unworthy of his wonderful healing power. However, this was just one of the many times HE would intervene on my behalf. During the next few years I had many catheterizations and heart procedures. I had earned the title of "heart patient", and I wasn't even fazed.

From 1989 to 1993, I had a few episodes with my heart which landed me in various hospitals for tests, catheterizations and stents. Doctors were always looking for a way to "fix" my heart, but it basically ended up doing the same thing over and over. It never dawned upon me that I was just "buying time" with each procedure. God was always faithful to see that I recovered in "record breaking" time and allowed me to get on with my life. I always felt that because of good doctors and a strong body, I would recover regardless of any procedure performed—and I usually did... BUT GOD! My part time service to HIM continued, but his response to me was 100%. I will say that as far as changing my life spiritually or becoming closer to him, it did not happen. These were just casual occurrences; God intervened, and Danny was not changed.

Chapter 4

The next major "scare" was in 1993 in Greenville, North Carolina. Again, while working on my job, I experienced traditional "angina/heart pains." They were so bad that I found myself lying on a stack of drywall trying to alleviate the pain. They did not go away so I contacted my cardiologist. He felt I needed another catheterization to see what was going on. It was scheduled, and I casually walked into the hospital for a procedure that I felt would be the same as so many before. It quickly turned into something much more serious. What started as a heart catherization whereby a stent would open the blockage was quickly changed to emergency bypass surgery. Two main arteries were completely blocked and could not be opened with a stent. Bypass was the only fix at this time. The doctors met with Peggy for consent for this surgery, and the procedure began. This spoke volumes to us because we began to realize that we were moving into a different territory as far as "heart recovery" and knew that this surgery had put us into a different category. I spent several days recovering, changing my diet, making new resolutions to change my lifestyle, and then like always… I recovered 100% and was soon back to my old way of working and going non stop. Not once did I experience a spiritual renewal that would open my eyes to see how God had protected me. I never had thoughts that I might die and that with this surgery it could have been the end. I am so sorry that I am now just seeing how God was speaking to me, trying to change me, but my ears and heart were definitely closed. Bypass surgery and a heart that can't be fixed with stents was soon in my rear view mirror.

Chapter 5

It was Saturday, July 2007, Wanchese, North Carolina, and Peggy and I had just returned from having lunch in Wanchese. I had felt perfectly ok up to that time but suddenly began to feel sharpening pains in my chest. I immediately became concerned because the pain was so unusually sharp and breathtaking. I told Peggy what I was experiencing and that I was going to lie down. She agreed that I should and if they got worse, we would go to the Outer Banks Hospital. It wasn't very long that I knew this was different. I told Peggy to take me at once, and we couldn't waste any time. She drove me to the hospital and on a Saturday on the Outer Banks of North Carolina in the summertime, that is quite a drive. We stopped for no lights, no traffic, and I felt for the first time that we may be too late getting there. I had never thought I was facing death before, but that day I was scared. I was bent over with pain and later was told I was having the "widowmaker"...the heart attack of all heart attacks. Thank God, we did arrive at the ER in time. Doctors and nurses began assisting me, and they soon realized that they could not help me. To them, it looked hopeless, and they told us they were air lifting me to Greenville. They gave us no hope that we'd even make it to the ER in Greenville, N.C. As they loaded me on the helicopter, I remember saying to Peggy and Cara..."I love you all." They both later said they felt they had seen me for the last time. As I stop now to think about how we were able to get to the OBX hospital and to the Greenville Heart Center, I am again made aware that MY GOD was in control. He had intervened again, and HE was not ready for me to die. I wasn't too sure about that at that time. I can tell you today that HE wanted to do a work in my life, but that wouldn't take place until 2019. Did I recognize this at that time? Absolutely not! He had already brought me out of two "life threatening" situations; this was just another intervention by the miraculous hand of GOD that I took for granted. I am so thankful that HIS timing is perfect.

Within the hour around 8:00 p.m. I had arrived at the Greenville Heart Center, and the doctors were standing by to begin working on me. At this point I was pretty much out of it but knew they were working frantically and got a sense that things might not be so good. Peggy had arrived from the Outer Banks and really did not know if I was dead or alive. That night the doctors discovered that my left ventricle was completely blocked. When they tried to open it, my heart stopped beating. Although I was not aware of what was going on, my family was notified that I was in trouble. Again, things looked very hopeless. I later heard from the doctors that they had used the "paddles" three times to bring me back and start my heart again. Now that explains the soreness and pain I felt when I woke up. The doctors were successful in opening the arteries in this left ventricle that night and keeping me alive. This was definitely a major Code Blue, but GOD was in charge, and Danny was just along for the ride.

The second morning in the hospital, I was visited in my spirit by what I believe to be an angel of the Lord. You may doubt or argue the fact of "who" this visitor was, but I am convinced that this visitor was from God. I was alone in the hospital. I had had a horrible night not only with pain and discomfort but also with mental torment of what was really going on, and if I was going to live. I was experiencing doubt like never before. Every other heart incident had happened, and I had recovered. This was different. I felt it in my soul. It was exactly 6:00 a.m. because I remembered the hands on the clock were straight up and down. I heard without a doubt a voice say to me: "AS YOUR SOUL PROSPERS, SO SHALL YOUR HEALTH." At first, I was terrified. I did not know at the time where it was in the Bible, but I thought it sounded like a scripture I had heard before. I later found it in 3rd John: 1:2. "Beloved, I wish above all things that thou mayest prosper and be in health, even as your soul prospers." The scripture was very easy for me to comprehend, but why was I hearing it on this particular morning? My health was certainly in terrible condition, and I had no idea what had even occurred the night before. All I knew was that I felt like a fallen, destitute individual who was completely out of control of his life. As I lay in bed that morning and thought about what the Lord had said to me, hope and faith began to rise. Maybe my health would be restored and with God's help, my body would get better. It seemed like an easy assignment...not really asking something impossible. I could do this! I was in church all the time leading worship and teaching. I knew how to get in contact with God. I'd just rededicate my life and commit myself to do more for him, and Danny would go on living. Sadly unchanged. I had been lying in bed all morning unable to move or even try to get up. I wasn't sure of my limitations because I had not spoken with the doctors. The staff was still very quiet. Peggy arrived at the hospital, and we were anxiously awaiting a report from the doctors. It seemed to be a very long morning, and we were hearing nothing. Around 2:00 p.m. my brother, Charlie, came to visit and check on how I was doing. We had a wonderful time visiting and talking about every subject under the sun, mainly construction. Of course, my mind was questioning if I would ever be able to work again. I had always bounced back... this was no different. Right? I needed answers. As Charlie was getting ready to leave, he asked me if I felt like getting out of bed and taking a walk. I had not been up since my surgery, and I told him that I wasn't sure that I should do it, much less even try to do it. My strength was gone, I had no energy, and I was fearful of even moving my body. Something impressed me to try. I told him I would walk with him; however, he would probably have to assist me. He did not have a problem with that so he helped me up, and we started out. I could hardly believe it! We walked around the hallway twice, and I had no problem at all. GOD HAD DONE WHAT HE SAID HE WOULD DO AT 6 a.m. The moment was very memorable. No one can say that the ANGEL OF THE LORD did not speak to me, and HE fulfilled his promise to me. In a very short time, I soon checked out of the hospital and returned to work. I did not forget the words I heard that morning...they rang in my ears daily, and I set out trying to change myself. I learned very quickly that God is the one who changes us, and we cannot do it within ourselves. Being so involved with working and the things of this world, my vision and passion that I felt in the hospital were soon dimmed. Danny was back to his old self. My life was prospering, but it was not prospering spiritually. The message that had spoken to my heart in the hospital seemed to fade with the passage of time. God had been faithful to restore my soul AGAIN. As I write today, I almost become angry with myself because it is now I sense the seriousness of what He wanted to do in my life. My plans were obviously more important so again I returned to living life with Danny in control.

Chapter 6

From 2008-2018, I experienced more heart issues due to calcium blockage. I had many catheterizations over the next ten years and a total of twelve stents. It was becoming a very "common" problem to me whether it was angina or terrific heart/chest pains. Thankfully, GOD had been in charge of my life, allowing me to always get to the hospital in time and get the attention and help I needed. It was just a way of life. I cannot tell you that it was because of my faithfulness to God or anything I had done for him. If my health depended on that, I would not be here to tell you. Oh, I can't name the times that I failed him, but he never failed me. My soul was not prospering as the scripture had instructed, but God never punished me for not living up to his instruction. I was learning to live with a severely damaged heart, and these close calls were just a norm. I became more relaxed with each procedure, and it just didn't scare me any more. My wonderful cardiologist in Greenville was always available to make sure I was getting the best treatment in spite of my careless living. I smile now when I reflect on our conversations and his desire to make me well. I'm sure he was frustrated at the casual way I approached all these incidents. My commitment to God the morning after my heart attack was long forgotten, and I was not changed.

Chapter 7

The next big "life threatening event" was on January 10, 2018 at St. Dominic Hospital in Jackson, Mississippi. While working as a construction supervisor, I began experiencing the traditional chest pains and shortness of breath that I had experienced so many times before. I knew I was in trouble...again. I went to a local cardiologist in Jackson and immediately found myself admitted to the Heart Center at this hospital. I was soon told that a catheterization needed to be done, and it had been scheduled for the next morning.

I had been in Jackson, MS six months building a church so I had no family with me. My doctors in Greenville were instrumental in finding the best cardiologist in Mississippi, and I am forever grateful. As you will read later, this doctor was certainly the right one at the right time. He had been hand picked by God. I called Peggy in NC and told her the plan. She immediately made plans to fly to Jackson that night thinking it would be our usual trip to the operating room. She arrived at midnight and was there for the catheterization the next morning. When the doctors completed that catheterization, they found that I had major heart blockage. These were the arteries that were used in my former bypass surgery in 1993. They could not open the blockage the usual way due to so many stents obstructing the entrance. The decision was made to try again the next day using a new procedure called IMPELLA 2.5. We knew nothing about this procedure, and the doctors confessed that they had only done twelve at that hospital; however, they had been successful. That alone was reason for concern. Due to the seriousness and possibility that this might not work, the doctors suggested if we had family that we should "get them there."

My daughter, Cara, left North Carolina immediately and flew to Jackson, Mississippi. Carolyn, Peggy's sister, and her husband, Jody, came from Dallas. Peggy had called them and spoken about the severity of this next catheterization. The doctors gave no hope other than saying it would be their best effort, and they had to try. If the blockage was not opened, I would die. They also explained to us that the IMPELLA 2.5 was a miniaturized, catheter-based intravascular blood pump that supports a patient's circulatory system. It provides continuous forward flow to the aorta to increase overall cardiac output, unload work from the ventricle, and improve coronary flow. Using this pump, the doctors hoped to be able to go in and clear these blockages. The risks were many, but the greatest one was not surviving this procedure. My family was given no hope. While we were waiting for "surgery time," Carolyn, my sister-in-law from Dallas, came to my bed and declared that God was in control and that HE was the healer. I am telling you she touched Heaven, and you could feel the presence of the Healer. She was convinced that everything would be ok, and I think she even convinced me too. We had a wonderful time of prayer and many tears. I believe everyone in that room realized that "nothing was impossible with God," and we would witness a miracle that day. Our faith was very strong. Even though I knew that I had failed God so many times, I was assured that He loved me and cared for me more than I could imagine. I could again go into this surgery with the confidence that I was in his hands. Our little prayer meeting had done wonders for my faith that day. The time came , and I was once again in surgery. All during the surgery the doctors would call Peggy and say, "He's still alive, but we aren't in. Keep praying." My crowd of prayer warriors would continue to pray and believe until they finally got the call... "We are in, it is open, and Danny is alive." Peggy says that when the doctors came out to speak to them, they looked like they'd been in a fight. They were physically worn out and exhausted. They told my family it was one of the most difficult things they had done. Peggy and Carolyn began to thank the doctors. Their response was, "Oh no...we didn't do this. We do not deserve the credit." Pointing Heavenward, they said, "A higher power did this surgery. We were only instruments." Again...God had a plan for me, and the Holy Spirit was there to see that it was carried out. I had survived another close call and my Sweet Jesus had brought me through. Having Christian doctors who told me they had asked God to guide their hands was just one of many miracles that day. Oh, how I praise HIM. After the experience in Jackson, I knew for sure that I was no longer a normal "heart patient" with a bad heart; I was a "heart patient" with a "severely damaged heart," and I was probably running out of time. I cannot comprehend why or how I have been blessed by God. My spirit was definitely moved by God's intervention that day, but to say I was changed spiritually would be a stretch. I also reflected on the scripture HE had given to me in 2007. I had prospered in many ways, but had I prospered spiritually? I momentarily took inventory of the past twenty years and thought of all the close calls I had had and all the times I had survived. Life has a way of moving on and so did I. I was thankful for what God had done, but I had work to do, a family to provide for, and goals I wanted to accomplish. I said my prayers thanking God and moved on. As I write this today, I am sick to my stomach as I look at how I took advantage of the goodness of God.

Chapter 8

I was scheduled to meet with my heart doctors in Greenville, NC in October 2018. They were aware of the procedure done in Jackson, MS and had kept in contact with those doctors. The meeting was to discuss a future plan for me since I had just about exhausted all that the regular cardiologist could do. I was referred to the "Heart Failure Clinic" the next month and boy, was this a real eye opener. The words "heart failure" should have been a good indication of where I was physically, but I don't think it sank in. I was told that stents, catheterizations, and all the other procedures that had "worked" for me in the past would no longer be an option. My heart was damaged, weak, and my blood flow was minimal. The ejection fraction is the percentage of blood in the heart that is pumped out with each heartbeat. A warning sign that you might be at risk of sudden cardiac arrest is if your ejection fraction is 35% or less. Mine was at 20% which is not supplying my heart with the blood that I needed. This was serious...we had to talk about other options.

At the next appointment in January 2019 we discussed the possibility of the LVAD (left ventricle assist device) surgery. A heart transplant was not an option because of my age and heart deterioation. I had no knowledge of this surgery, but I did know my heart was weakening with each day. I was continuing to work but was noticing shortness of breath almost daily. Had I waited too late to get the help I needed? Would I survive this "unknown" surgery? I thought of my family's DNA and the many that had experienced heart problems, including my great grandfather who died at 38 with a bad heart. My uncles and my father also had experienced problems with their hearts. It seemed this gene had certainly been passed down to me. Up to this point, you could say I was hardheaded, but I can tell you after meeting with these doctors to discuss my options, I was thinking more seriously now. I listened to all they had to say in that meeting. They had my attention for a short while and then I traveled home from Greenville, NC. The next day I got on a plane to go to my job in California. Far away from home... living alone, and working everyday. That certainly doesn't define someone worried about his heart giving out. Obviously, I had listened to what they said, but I had not heard a word they were saying.

January 30 I was on a job in California, and I received a call from the Heart Failure Clinic advising me to come in for another consultation. This time they emphasized the point that I could be running out of time. It was imperative that I consider this LVAD surgery; it was my only option, and it needed to be done very soon. Again, I was not able to understand the magnitude of my heart problem. I found myself meeting with a team of doctors on February 12th and 13th, 2019 to further discuss my LVAD options. Peggy and I had to be "schooled" in the procedure, the danger, the maintenance and all the other one hundred effects it could have. It was so unknown to us, but when you only have one option left, what do you do?

This operation would take a total commitment. We would have to meet with many doctors to sign off to show that we were mentally capable of going through this procedure. This checkout was required by the hospital and insurance companies. The doctors believed we were good candidates and so the plan was set in action. I was going to be scheduled for the LVAD surgery. I had no other choice. Vidant Hospital had not done a lot of these surgeries, and that was a big concern for us. Were we able to trust this hospital and these doctors? Bottom line...we had to, and we were smart enough to know that God would be present, and we trusted Him for the outcome. It is easy to get spiritual in a time like this. I found myself convincing God that my soul had really prospered, and I knew He would bring me through this. Of course, HE knew better.

I will interject here that this surgery would have been impossible without Peggy's support. One person could never take this on...it is definitely a team effort.

Chapter 9

Since we were already in Greenville, I was admitted to the hospital on the 14th, hopefully for a heart catheterization and to check pressures in my heart. This would be the basic procedure before final approval was given that we were perfect candidates. That procedure showed again my heart ejection fraction was at 20%; basically, not pumping enough blood to keep me alive. I had planned to go home after this procedure, but the doctors said if I left the hospital, I would not live. My heart was too weak, and something had to be done immediately. Of course, we stayed in the hospital and on February 20th the Heart Failure Team felt the only option left for me was to have the LVAD surgery. Not really knowing how all of this would work, we received a crash course from the team. We had multiple doctors, nurses, and coordinators coming in constantly giving us mini lessons on what was going to take place and the risks involved. To say our brains were in overload is an understatement. We even had calls from "friends" telling us to reconsider Greenville Hospital and go to Duke or Chapel Hill. Several times we felt like we had Job's advisors. We watched surgeries on YouTube, read pamphlets, spoke with one person who had had this surgery, and tried our hardest to comprehend what was about to take place. Basically, this is a pump attached to the heart to keep the left ventricle open and the blood flowing. The pump is controlled by electricity and batteries. The patient must wear a controller and two five-pound batteries at all times to generate power to the pump. The controller is like a computer and records blood flow, pump speed, pulse index, and pump power. It is something that you must look at very often to make sure the numbers and alarms are what they should be. A driveline leads from an open incision that has been made in the stomach. The cord runs from the heart to the controller, along with two battery cables. These cables are always connected to batteries and must be charged daily. They cannot get wet or damaged. The incision that is made on the stomach has the driveline coming from the heart and must be cleaned and those bandages changed weekly. You may think this was easy to comprehend, but there is no way to tell you how impossible it was to understand. It isn't normal...it is hard...it is awkward. This was going to be a life changing event and there is no way to understand it prior to the surgery. It would change everything about me; the way I dressed...the way I bathed...my daily activities...every detail of my life. I was listening to all of this, but again I was not hearing. To say that we were in the dark was an understatement. What should we do? We had been told that my life would end very quickly if we didn't try this procedure. I thought of my wife, Peggy; my daughter, Cara; and her kids, Ragen and Spencer. There are no words to tell you how much I love them. I wanted to live for them...see Ragen and Spencer graduate from college and go on to have families of their own. I wanted to see them serving God and becoming what HE had planned for them. Putting my family in this perspective, the decision was becoming very clear. Knowing we had two options, life or death, we chose to trust GOD and the doctors, and we gave our consent. Yes, we would go ahead and do this.

Surgery was scheduled for February 21, 2019.

Knowing this day would change my life forever, I felt it necessary that the doctors understood what I wanted from this surgery. Would my quality of life improve or would I sit in a rocker the rest of my days? Would I work? Would I be able to live a normal life connected with ten pounds of batteries? I wanted more than just being able to breathe, and they assured me that a successful surgery would not only extend my life but give me a good quality of life. I can not tell you today that I understood the medical side of this surgery. I just know I was convinced that it was the right thing to do. Three years and eight months later I stand by my decision.

Chapter 10

That night before surgery I was only thinking of surviving. Everyone had left; I was alone. I began to think about what was getting ready to happen the next day. My mind was spinning. My life and independence were about to change. Questions flooded my mind, and no answers were available. I had never had this feeling of being so alone in all the years I had been in the hospital. I was most confident that the Heavens were brass and the God who spoke to me in 2007 was just not available or interested in hearing my plea. I had certainly not kept any bargain that I had made in prior surgeries or hospital visits so why would God be attentive to me tonight. The enemy was doing all he could do to magnify my failures and unfaithfulness and almost had me convinced that calling out to God would be a wasted effort. I had been in church all of my life…sixty-eight years. As I stated before, I had served as associate pastor and worship leader. I had encouraged others so many times to "take their burdens to the Lord" and that He would turn their situations around. Now the shoe was on the other foot. I needed to pray, and words would not come. This was the time to have a conversation with God. This was critical, and I needed to have his peace at this moment. I was forgetting to "come to the throne room of God" with BOLDNESS as my Heavenly Father had instructed us to do. I felt very awkward. I did not feel like His son. I knew God to be more than able to grant my requests, but on the other hand, I knew my shortcomings. The evil one knew them too, and this was a perfect time for him to fill my head with negative thoughts. He told me I deserved nothing from God because of my failures, my unkept promises, and my lack of dedication to God. This was a perfect time to bring up my past and all my weaknesses, and he did! I actually felt the oppression from the enemy, and I needed peace from my Savior. I did what I had instructed so many others to do, and what I knew I needed to do at this moment. I just began to pray a very simple prayer asking God that "His will be done." I felt my words were inadequate, and I needed to pray more sophisticatedly. My heart was faithless, and I could sense that I was getting nowhere. All my biblical teaching was beginning to fall short; I was searching for peace and real life answers. I rolled and tossed all night praying, thinking, and knowing that if I could touch God, I would be able to go into surgery with a "peace that passeth understanding." Feeling hopeless in my praying, I immediately quit trying to impress God and just simply asked again for His will and favor. I had no more energy to perform any special tricks to merit his grace. I just approached his throne and asked very humbly. It was in HIS hands now. The enemy would have to taunt someone else… I had come as a child, and I realized God expected nothing but just my heart…a simple plea to him. He was waiting and ready. His peace flooded my soul, and I was soon asleep.

Chapter 11

The next five days after the LVAD surgery would be lessons that would take me three and a half years to comprehend. As I tell you about my experience during those five days, I will be the first to admit that this experience is one that I relive every day of my life. I do not understand all that happened, but I do recognize the change that has taken place in my life. I did not see a light or other things that some people have experienced. I did have what I describe for lack of words an "out of body experience." My hope is that I can relate to you what God did in my life during those "after surgery" days. I was transformed during this experience, and I want to share it so that you, the reader, can too experience what God desires to do in all of us. If I had known as I lay alone that night of what God was going to do in my life, I would have been so joyful. Instead, I temporarily let the enemy almost rob me of realizing that God had a plan for me, and it was getting ready to unfold. The plan that HE started in my life as a child was getting ready to be revealed. I am saddened that I wasted so much of my life being in control. I ask God to forgive me. Well, I am jumping ahead, but let's go back to the day of surgery.

February 21st I was scheduled for LVAD HEARTMATE 3 surgery at Vidant Hospital in Greenville, NC. The nurses and staff prepared me, and I was on my way. Knowing that my surgeon had done several of these operations at Duke and Greenville, I felt the confidence and trust that he was the best one to do this even though all of this was new to me. I smile as I think back that I didn't even know enough about the surgery to ask him any questions. Prior to the operation he asked if I had any questions. My reply to him was, "Doc, just do your best." I had a brief time with my family and then the anesthesiologist came in and did the last preparation. It was around 11:00 that morning.

My life was completely out of my control at that point, and God was beginning to pick up where I had left off. What an incredible journey this was going to be.

Chapter 12

My family was in the waiting room not knowing the outcome of this day. They were not hearing anything from the doctors, and I can't imagine the anxiety they were having.

Peggy, my daughter Cara, and my sister, Flora, were in for the long haul, and I am sure it was not an easy day. They received updates during the day but nothing that gave them hope that this surgery was going to be a success. Around 9:00 p.m. the surgeon came out to speak with them. They said he, too, looked frazzled and like he had been in a fight. He appeared exhausted and very worried. He made the comment to them that I must be a "bionic man on steroids" because of the difficulty of cutting through the calcium buildup and the numerous stents in my heart. He gave the good news that the pump was attached successfully to the heart and was working. The concern now was blood flow and how my body would react to this foreign object. Because the doctors needed to monitor this pump and my blood flow for twenty-four hours, I was left open. My chest was exposed so that they could watch the blood flow, look for excessive bleeding and to make it easier if they needed to go back in. I had been "packed" with sterile foam to absorb the unnecessary bleeding. Precaution was taken so that blood clots did not develop. After the doctor had "schooled" the family in what had taken place, he made the comment that "we are not out of the woods, and I cannot tell you that Danny will survive this." He was hesitant to call the surgery a success at this point and even said it was one of the top five worst surgeries he had ever done. Of course, the family was exhausted, fearful, and certainly not wanting to hear this. Around 10:00 or so they were invited into the recovery room to see me. I was unconscious, and they were not able to talk to me. I am sure it relieved their minds just to know that this day was over but knowing we could not call this a success yet, they left the recovery room very distraught. Immediately they met my former cardiologist who had been with the surgery team checking on my progress. I had been his patient for many years until he referred me to the Heart Failure Clinic. Being the wonderful, caring doctor that he is, he wanted to be there for this procedure. He, too, looked very tired and worried, and told my family to "keep praying." Hopelessness was exactly what they said they were feeling and knew that only God could complete this task. They began to call prayer chains and the saints of the Church to pray. We needed a miracle and we knew exactly where to go to ask for it. We had seen God work many times before, and this night was no different. Knowing that people were praying gave hope and confidence to the family after a very long exhausting day.

Chapter 13

The family continued to pray and wait while I was in the recovery room. There is no way for me to explain to you what was getting ready to take place in the next five days because I certainly had no clue. These days would teach me so much about the Trinity: God the Father, God the Son, and God the Holy Spirit. I had been taught that I was created in the image of God...Body, Soul, and Spirit. I was about to experience this in real time. I am going to try to convey to you where God took me during those days. I hope I can do it justice. I had an "out of body experience" and no one can change my mind. My family tells me I was out for five days and it was during this time that I was visited by what I believe was an angel of the Lord and the Holy Spirit. I am using the five days as a time reference because the experience seemed to happen in segments. I was taken to a place where my soul and mind were transformed, and my life was changed. These days after surgery…five days unconscious would be the worst of my life but the best of my life. These days have changed me so much that I am even amazed at myself. The greatest part of this operation was not what was done for my heart but what was done in my life spiritually.

Chapter 14

On day one of my unconsciousness, February 21st, I was visited by what I believe was an angel of the Lord and the Holy Spirit. The angel did not speak to me, but took my soul and spirit out of my physical body. I could look down and see my body lying on the table as the angel led me out of the room. It seemed I was taken to a "future" time and place. I had no clue what was going on, but my physical man had been left behind, and I was traveling with an angel who was saying nothing to me. The angel and Holy Spirit would rocket me forward in time to the war between Good and Evil...the war between the saints and the sinner. I had read about this in the Bible and heard about it all of my life. I will never forget this encounter. Scared to death is an understatement. The teaching class by the angel would soon begin without a word even spoken. Remember, my physical body is unconscious, left in the operating room. I always thought if you were unconscious that the total man was asleep. This was not so with me. I was having a meeting with an angel and the Holy Spirit, and they were leading me to some place. There is no way for me to explain days with my soul and my spirit. When I call a day, I am speaking of the 24 hour time frame that we as humans know. That's the only way I can even try to explain it. I found myself up on a mountain looking down at a huge valley where destruction was taking place.

There was definitely a battle going on. I saw fire, brimstone, jets flying, people being killed and forces fighting against one another. I heard screaming and crying, and I knew that this was a picture of HELL that I had heard about as a child. I can not describe this because my vocabulary is too limited. I do know that it was horrible, and I was shaking with fear. The angel left me on that mountain, and I was alone. I stood and watched these terrible events and to this day, I can not get them out of my mind.

Chapter 15

I was still unconscious on day two. Remember, I am thinking in 24-hour periods since my experience took place in segments at different places. This is the only way I can explain my journey. I remained on the mountain top where the angel and Holy Spirit had left me, and I was witnessing things that are indescribable. I thought that I might have been left in Hell, and my soul was tormented by this thought. I am there, but was I to stay here in this place? Is God turning His back on me now? I thought I was a good person. Did I deserve Hell? Was this the end? There are no words to describe the hopelessness and regret that I was feeling. I realize now that the war I saw was the one written about in Revelation of a war to come—the Great Battle between good and evil. I had heard in church about a "battle" that would be fought in the end time. At that moment, I couldn't comprehend that this was what I was seeing. I felt very much a part of this. When I felt I could not stand another second of this destruction, the angel appeared to me a second time. You can just imagine how happy I was to see the angel. I immediately spoke to the angel by quoting a scripture that I knew most of my life. Maybe if the angel heard me quote a scripture, I would be led away from this place. I quoted Romans 10:9, "If thou shalt confess with thy mouth the Lord Jesus, and shalt believe in thine heart that God hath raised him from the dead, thou shalt be saved." I wanted this angel to know that I had confessed with my mouth and I did believe. Still saying nothing to me, the angel soon left. What? I was going to be left here again after I had quoted scripture and expressed my belief in God. I was alone and still scared as ever on this huge battlefield. The fighting and destruction continued as I watched fearfully. I was at the end; I could take no more. My physical body was still hanging between life and death. I had no clue what was going on in that hospital, but I can tell you I was experiencing Hell.

While back at the hospital, the doctors were working very hard to save my life. The surgery wasn't finished. The doctors were beginning to remove the sterile foam and to close my chest, like bypass surgery. That evening before Peggy went to the motel, the doctors allowed her to see me.

She and other family members came in and prayed over me before they left for the night. This was something they did every night while I was in the hospital. I could not hear them, but I'm mighty glad they were praying. If they had just had a clue where I was. They were seeing this pitiful physical body, but I was not there. They were on a wait and pray plan. My physical body was in a deep sleep, but my soul and spirit were watching a great battle take place. Was this the Battle of Armageddon? According to the Book of Revelation in the New Testament, Armageddon is the prophesied location of a gathering of armies for a battle during the end times. I knew enough of past teaching that Revelation does tell of a final war—when and how it begins, who lives and who dies. What I was seeing was unbelievable. I do not know if I was seeing this particular battle, but I do know that I witnessed great destruction and killing, and I was scared beyond words. The only thing that I am sure of is that the angel took me to a time in the future. I was alone, scared, but the sights I saw were off the charts. I shall never forget. Obviously my quoting the scripture did not impress the angel. I was concentrating on myself... I really don't think I was cooperating with the Holy Spirit on why I had been brought to this place. Not yet, anyway. If I had made an impression on the angel, it certainly did not change my location.

Chapter 16

The next day as I again refer to as our 24-hour day was February 23rd. The physical person was still in the balances of life and death. The doctors were at my side working with various medical problems and the adjustments of the new pump. The family continued in the waiting room for another day. I still had the breathing tube in and all the other machines hooked up. What amazed me was that the physical man could not move, hear, see, or feel anything. The soul and spirit were on a journey that I perceived to be Hell. I wanted so badly to leave this place.

At some point the angel made another visit to the horrible high hill or mountain that I had been agonizing on for the last hours. As usual, the angel did not speak to me but just stood beside me. I was very aware of a "presence" and so happy to see this heavenly being again. I spoke to the angel. This time I quoted my favorite verse Isaiah 43:1 "But now this saith the Lord that created thee, O Jacob and he that formed thee, O Israel, fear not: for I have redeeemed thee, I have called thee by thy name; thou art mine." Like before, my verse of scripture did not impress the angel of the Lord. She remained silent as together we continued watching the action on the battlefield. It was just getting worse, and Hell seemed very close. Quoting my scripture had not changed my situation at all. What could I do or say to be able to leave this place? I did not know if my physical body was dead or alive, and I certainly did not understand the purpose of this encounter. Have I died on the operating table and been sent to Hell? The degree of torment was unbelievable. The angel must have thought I needed more time in this awful place to observe, reflect, and examine myself. After all my broken promises to God, was the angel making sure I was getting the point? Could I stand to be in this place another 24 hours? With this level of fear and torment, I could not imagine the stress that my heart was experiencing. The stress that I was experiencing in my soul and spirit was almost more than I could handle. I had really messed up things, and now God was having the last word with me. Hell is real, and I had seen it first hand.

Every day Peggy and family stayed at the hospital and would always come by my bed at night to pray. Oh, how I needed them to know where I was so that they could really touch God to get me out of this place. I was fearful that it was too late for me.

Not much changed during the day, but I was stable. God was working miracles in my body, and doctors were becoming hopeful. If only I could have had just a glimmer of hope as I was on the mountain top. The angel had left me again and I was beginning to doubt my entire relationship with God. At this point it was evident that I was lost and doomed for Hell. The angel had come to me, left me at the brink of Hell, and I was terrified. I had lost all hope that the angel would return and take me away from this place. I then had feelings of wanting to die and end it all. I could not take another minute of this. If I'm doomed for Hell then let it happen and stop this uncertainty. I didn't know what the angel or the Holy Spirit was doing, but I was ready to stop this foolishness. If God did not intervene, it was over, and it certainly did not look like that was going to happen.

Chapter 17

The next day in my time, February 24th, things began to turn around. My situation with my heart is better, and the family is feeling hopeful. The best part that I experienced is that the angel appeared to me on the mountain. The angel took me by the hand, and we moved from that horrible hell of the war between good and evil to a place in my past. To tell you how relieved I was would take the entire English language. I was taken to a little church where my father was pastoring in Wanchese, North Carolina. I was just a little boy about six years old sitting in my Sunday school class listening to my teacher tell us about Jesus. The teacher was singing "Jesus Loves Me" and we children were singing along. The words continued by saying, "Jesus Loves me because the Bible tells me so." I knew that I had experienced the love of God as a child and His love is forever. He loves me! I am not in Hell. I am being reminded that Jesus loves me and oh, what a sweet message to hear. I had been so afraid and full of torment. Now I was beginning to feel a peace that maybe "all was well." Not anything I had done but simply His love for me. I hardly had time to take this moment in before the angel very quickly took me by the hand again to another destination. I was not worried about my physical body or wondering if I had made it or not. The peace that I was experiencing was so wonderful that I just wanted to stay in this place. The angel had a different agenda. This time we were standing in front of a huge gate with flashing red lights with the written word REDEEMED. One moment I was standing at the brink of Hell knowing that I was doomed for eternity, and now I see the gates of Heaven shouting REDEEMED. I was so excited. I began to look for the lights of Heaven...If I see a crack, I'm going in, but that was not the plan. My excitement was almost more than I could contain. The peace and love that I was feeling were overwhelming and now...just now, I may be entering the gates of Heaven. This is just too much for one to comprehend. I did not want it to end. As I was planning my strategy to slip through those beautiful gates, I realized the angel had a different plan. That night she took me back so that I could see my physical body, but my soul and spirit remained with the angel. I could see my hands, my feet, my eyes...but I could not communicate with my physical body. I was just seeing myself...nothing else.

Remember, my family is continuing to come in every night and pray with me. They have picked up nurses who asked to join them in prayer. What a wonderful witness. Oh, how I hope that they witnessed the powerful hand of God as the family prayed each night for my recovery.

Chapter 18

It is the 5th day of my unconsciousness, February 25th, and I am totally exhausted.

My soul and spirit are very tired and my body is equally tired. Very soon the angel would visit me for our final encounter to let me know the love that Jesus has for me. Believe me, I was ready for some good news and a declaration that "my soul was saved." Very soon I would be persuaded that I am the apple of his eye, and that nothing can separate me from the love of God. Romans 8: 38, "For I am persuaded that neither death, nor life, nor angels, nor principalities, nor power, nor things present, nor things to COME..." Yes, I had witnessed what was coming, but I did not need to fear. Bottom line... nothing can separate us from the love of God. For us to understand the love of God we have to understand the fact that God loves us just the way we are. Yes, with all our scars and brokenness and baggage...He loves us. I felt the presence of the angel and the Holy Spirit, and I knew that I was in the presence of God. After what I had seen and encountered, this was such a sweet place to be. My soul and spirit began to talk to the angel. I started by saying I wanted to love God more than anything in my life. I also wanted to love my family more than myself, and last of all, I wanted to love every person with whom I came in contact. For this to happen I had to start by fixing the only person I could fix: ME. All my life when I had a problem with someone I would try to tell them how they could be better, and the changes they needed to make. After my encounter with the angel, I realized I just needed to fall in love with Jesus, and He would change me. 2 Corinthians 5:17, " Therefore if anyone is in Christ, he is a new creation." Now that's a definite change, and I wanted it. I noticed now that the angel had left, and I was back in my body. I remained unconscious to everyone else.

Peggy told me that the doctors started to take the tubes out that day. The last one to come out would be the breathing tube; however, they had to make sure I was able to breathe on my own. Timing is everything, and it was very soon that my oxygen level was stable. My major organs were not rejecting the pump. The pump speed was set in relation to my body, and it was doing its job without any problems.

I was taking quite a bit of medicine, and my body was cooperating with that also. I was moving right along. I was still unconscious, but very much aware of the finality of the angel's visit and all that had transpired. I was ready to live…to live for God.

Finally, in the afternoon the doctor came into the waiting room to get Peggy. They told her that I was coming too, and she should start talking to me. Peggy came into the recovery room and was very anxious that this moment had arrived. Her first words to me were, "Wake up, Danny Boy; you made it." I turned and looked at her and said, "Peggy, we cannot miss Heaven!" Thinking that I was probably still out of my head, she was a little taken back with that comment. I repeated this to her and she could see the seriousness in my eyes. She knew immediately that something had taken place in my life while I was unconscious. It would be several weeks before I would ever tell her all that happened. I knew that this story would be perceived as "unbelievable" to those who would hear it. I would have to trust God to reveal this experience to those who heard it. This I know…it was very real to me. She was a little surprised by my first comment because we had been in church all our lives and Heaven was certainly our final destination. Her reply was very nonchalant and she just casually said, "We aren't going to miss Heaven." I again was made aware that this will be a difficult story to tell. I became conscious very slowly because of the equipment and remaining necessary tubes. I could hardly talk or understand everything that was going on, but felt it necessary to tell her again. I said to her, "No, Peggy, we cannot miss Heaven." She heard my determination but had no clue why these would be my first words after five days. I had so much to tell her. I was alive. Now my body, soul, and spirit were together. I knew that the Holy Spirit was there, and I had been in the Presence of Jehovah, God Almighty, Prince of Peace. I would just have to enjoy this new love relationship, and in God's time I would tell my story, and people would believe it.

Chapter 19

As I recovered daily, I shared with Peggy my desire to love God, love her, and love people like I had never loved before. Although she had not heard any of my experience, she knew that something had happened. My spirit was sweeter; I was more gentle, and obviously not the same Danny who went into surgery on February 21, 2019. Everyone who visited noticed the change in me. I was so tender, and I welcomed the tears that would flow when I talked about how I loved Jesus. I lay in bed and just worshiped Him. I had experienced first hand his love for me. He did not want me to be destroyed or to go to Hell. He did everything he could so that I could be redeemed. My faith was renewed, and I enjoyed "practicing the presence of God." I did not share my experience with anyone; I was still trying to absorb what had happened, and I was just not ready to tell it. All I wanted to do was tell of the love of God, and I probably sounded like a broken record to those who came by.

The next few days the physical man had many questions. There was pain…so much equipment, lots of medicine, bags, and drips, and the maintenance for this pump was unbelievable. Being alive was working for me but definitely had many challenges. I experienced pneumonia and lung collapse around the 5th of March. Fluid was developing around my heart. They had to hook me up with a machine that would "shake" me vigorously trying to eliminate the fluid. Try having that done when your chest has been split open. So many after surgery experiences; however, I was constantly thinking about my "out of body" experience. It was real, and I was constantly going back to what I had witnessed. I knew that I had so many things to work on in my life, but right now, I was just enjoying living knowing how much God loved me.

I was trying to love and be peaceful, but it was difficult. For the first time in my life, I was experiencing stress and nervousness like never before. It still amazes me that the doctors did not see the need for my mind to be addressed with the magnitude of the surgery, medicine, maintenance of pump, and rehabilitation.

The healing process of this operation demanded total healing. If you looked at my physical body, you would think I was in almost perfect condition, responding well to the operation. No one could see my mental condition. Stress, nerves, sleep deprivation and anxiety all were wearing on me. Spiritually I was in the best shape, maybe a little overboard. All I wanted to talk about was God. I had my perspectives in the right order. There was no doubt that God would be first in my life from now on. This experience had not only frightened me, but it had changed me. I would not be the apathetic Christian that I had been before this experience.

My soul would prosper and this time it would be 100%.

Chapter 20

As challenges came with the acceptance of the pump, we found some of them to be overwhelming. I was now allergic to some of the medicine and unable to take them. Some of the meds affected my nerves which led to other problems. I did not want any noise, lights, or even people around me. People around me having conversations made me very edgy, and I just wanted darkness and quietness. This was partly medicine and partly adjusting to the foreign object in my body. Working through this was one of the hardest parts of the "after operation" experience. Also, the hospital was pushing me to have different kinds of rehab soon after the surgery. My nerves could not take all the adjustments that the staff was demanding me to go through; at times, I thought their demands were worse than the surgery. I was a basket case. Yes, I was alive, but my physical man was beyond miserable.

BUT GOD....another memorable experience. As my Heavenly Father, he knew I needed peace, and this came on a Saturday afternoon around 5:00 p.m.

Peggy was preparing to return home to Wanchese because she played the piano in a local church and needed to be there for Sunday morning. As she was packing up getting ready to leave and making sure I was set for the night, I asked her to do something special for me. I told her I needed to hear an old song that I remembered from my childhood. I could tell I was delaying her, and she wasn't very happy about it. She made the comment that my nerves would not allow me to tolerate any noise of any kind so hearing music was out of the question. I think she saw how important this was to me so she searched Youtube until she found the song I had requested. The song I wanted to hear was, "I Am Redeemed; Behold I Stand Amazed" by an artist whom I remember hearing as a child. My parents would play his long play albums at night, and I remember hearing this particular song many nights before falling asleep. God had brought this back to my memory and knew I needed it for this day. She found this specific song and lay the phone on my shoulder so that I could hear it clearly. Oh my...the music began, and I immediately felt the presence of the Holy Spirit. Peggy and I began to weep, pray, and worship. Oh, the joy of His presence...

again. As we were sitting in this room, just the two of us, listening and worshiping, the door of my room swung open. The doctor and several nurses rushed in. They asked, "What is going on here? And, you are crying." I said to him that these were tears of joy. He said, "Well, I believe in all of that, but your heart rate has spiked to 153 and that can't happen." One nurse even had a needle in her hand ready to give me a shot to bring down my heart rate. We stopped the music and waited for them to check me out. We all settled down, and they left the room. Peggy and I looked like two kids who had been caught with our hand in the cookie jar. We just laughed and laughed. What a precious moment we had experienced worshiping the one who has redeemed us.

On her way home, Peggy said she was in Columbia, NC, and was thinking about what had happened at the hospital. She said that she was laughing to herself at what had happened when she felt the Lord speak to her heart.

He asked, "How long has it been since your heart rate spiked at the mention of my name?" She said it hit her like a ton of bricks, and she began to cry and ask God to forgive her. She also felt him say to her, "Don't let your heart grow callused." We have thought of that experience so many times. What a powerful question to ask yourself. Just think about that. If we truly love God, shouldn't our hearts spike when we feel His glorious presence?

Chapter 21

Have you grown callused in your service to God? When I had the encounter with the angel and Holy Spirit during my unconsciousness, my life was changed drastically, and I did not even know what God was doing. The angel certainly was not communicating with me, but during that time God was working in my life. My stale, callused relationship has become one that desires to be in His presence every minute of every day. God changed me, and I will never be the same. If you desire a fresh start in your walk with God, allow Him to work in your life. No distractions from the evil one. Humble yourself, trust GOD and see his glory. He wants us to come as children, that six-year-old little boy. With all the baggage, scars, and wounds, GOD still wants you as you are. Quit trying to clean up your life. Your Heavenly Father will pick up the pieces and make something beautiful of your life. Love God and he will do the rest. You can be changed by seeking God. He is constantly pursuing you. Jeremiah 29:13: "And ye shall seek me, and find me, when ye shall search for me with all your heart." Yes, it is that simple, and we make it so difficult. I am so thankful that God has been patient with me for over thirty years. As I have written down all the things that I have experienced in this book, I am constantly amazed at God's mercy. I have been writing for several weeks about how God has intervened in my life with all these "heart incidents" but they were all planned by Him. He knew that each time he was preparing and molding me for this final surgery. He had my encounter with the angel and Holy Spirit planned all along. I cannot tell you how thankful I am for his patience with me. I certainly do not deserve it.

Chapter 22

With each day, I became more familiar with "my pump" and felt I was making progress as a patient. My stay in the hospital after surgery consisted of many different kinds of rehab and encounters with medical staff training me for the usage and protection of my equipment. It was an education within itself for Peggy and me. Peggy had to take a test on "knowing the LVAD pump" and had to demonstrate her knowledge in all parts of it. She also had to show how she could change the nightly bandages covering the incision. This is all important because no bacteria or germs can enter the driveline incision. Knowing the thirty-five pills and their function was also new to her. Of course, she passed with flying colors, and I felt confident that I was in good hands.

The doctors would come in daily to check on me. Each time I spoke with them I would thank them for what they had done but would also tell them that I knew God had brought me through this surgery. I did not hesitate to give all the glory to God. Maybe I was finally learning how God was and is in control of my life.

As I was preparing to go home from the hospital, the surgeon came in to tell me goodbye. Now, remember, each time I had spoken to him I had expressed my faith in God. He never seemed to respond or even believe. We talked about my health and how different life would probably be for me. I asked the surgeon if the LVAD team had any medical follow up that addressed one's mental position while in surgery. I had been unconscious for five days, and no one seemed to be interested in what may have happened while I was out. I had had a spiritual "out of the body" experience and no one knew anything about it. If there had been a psychiatrist or someone to speak with me about that, it would have been very helpful. He said that no one addressed the "mental" part of this surgery but agreed it was needed. I definitely agreed. When we said our goodbyes, he turned to leave the room. The next thing he said to me before leaving was "pray for me." He may not have had a tear in his eye, but I certainly did. Wow. I won't ever forget that wonderful man with such a wonderful heart.

Chapter 23

Growing up in a Christian home with a Christian family, I can say that God was the center of our lives. He has always been a part of my life even when I was not doing my part. As I reflect on the past thirty years, I am reminded of the miracles that He has performed in my life. This last encounter with Him during the LVAD surgery however was the greatest change that has ever taken place in my life. It has been a spiritual explosion for me. As I worked on this book daily for several months, I remembered the many times

God had been in control of my life. If not, I would not be here today to write about it. Surviving the operation physically was certainly a wonderful thing; however, it was not the purpose God had for me. It changed me spiritually and I am not the same person I was on February 21, 2019. I know first hand now of the love of Jesus... I went to him as a child and my life was changed. Would I do this over again? The answer is a thousand times YES! Knowing God is worth everything! I love the verse in 1 John 4:16, "We know how much God loves us, and we have put our trust in his love. God is love, and all who live in love live in God, and God lives in them."

I don't expect you, the reader, to understand all that I have attempted to write. Being visited by a heavenly being who never spoke to me, but took me to three different places is a stretch. As I have described these places to you, I am sure questions have filled your mind as I tried to relate them as they happened to me. I understand that. Each day I still relive these events and let them unravel in my mind again. Although I can't explain it...it happened, it changed me, and I am a different person.

Let me say one final word. Jesus is coming back, and I believe very soon. I am going to see him face to face, but "until that day my heart will go on singing." I shall sing of his love, his faithfulness, his mercy, and his Amazing Grace. Don't you want to know him? Romans 10:9, "If you confess with your mouth, 'Jesus is Lord,' and believe in your heart that God raised Him from the dead, you will be saved." LET HIM CHANGE YOUR LIFE TODAY. JUST ACCEPT HIM.

YOU SEE...WE JUST CAN'T MISS HEAVEN!

Psalm 103

"How could I ever forget the *miracles* of *kindness* you've done for me? You *kissed* my heart with *forgiveness*, in spite of all I've done.
You've *healed* me inside and out from every disease. You've *rescued* me from hell and *saved* my life. You've *crowned* me with love and mercy. You *satisfy* my every desire with good things. You've *supercharged* my life so that I *soar* again like a flying eagle in the sky!"